CONTENTS

INTRODUCTION

Mushrooms are adored around the world as food sources. Many species are used to give an earthy flavor and meaty texture to everything from pizza to risotto. But if you consume a certain type of mushrooms, that pizza will make your dining experience rather, well, magical. Known as magic mushrooms, shrooms, mushies, psychedelic mushrooms, psychotropic mushrooms or psilocybin, these mushrooms cause differences in mood, perception and behavior that are commonly known as "tripping." These types of mushrooms belong to the genus Psilocybe. Mushrooms of other genera can also cause hallucinations, but many purists insist that Psilocybe mushrooms are the "true" magic mushrooms. Psilocybe mushrooms cause hallucinations because they contain the psychotropic tryptamines psilocybin and psilocin (some species also contain other, weaker psychotropic compounds like baeocystin or norbaeocystin). A single mushroom contains anywhere from 0.1 to 1.3 percent psilocybin.

MAGIC MUSHROOM

Magic mushrooms are one of the most widely used recreational psychotropic drugs because they can be found in the wild or grown fairly easily and inexpensively. According to the 2018 National Survey on Drug Use and Health, about 1.3 percent of adults over the age of 26 in the United States had used hallucinogens in the past year (a category that includes LSD, mushrooms and MDMA, among other substances) [source: Substance Abuse & Mental Health Services Administration]. Unlike manufactured psychotropic drugs such as LSD, magic mushrooms have a long history dating back thousands of years as part of religious or spiritual ceremonies. However, magic mushrooms also have a lot in common with LSD. Let's start with looking at how eating them can affect people. Mushrooms have a lot in common with LSD in terms of how they affect the body. Both are psychotropic drugs and act on the central nervous system to produce their effects. Many people have described a mushroom trip as a milder, shorter version of an LSD trip. Like LSD, magic mushrooms don't technically cause hallucinations, or visions of things that aren't actually there. Instead, they distort the perception of actual objects.

People tripping on mushrooms might see things in different colors or see patterns. Existing colors, sounds, tastes and textures may be distorted, while feelings and emotions intensify. It can feel like time has sped up, slowed down or stopped completely. There can be a changed perception of one's place in the universe and a feeling of communing with a higher power. As with LSD, what happens on a mushroom trip varies by person, dosage and the type of mushroom eaten, as some are more powerful than others.

"Set and setting," or the emotional state of the user and the type of environment he or she is in, play a big part in whether the trip is positive. Users who are in a poor mental state or a highly structured environment are more likely to have a bad trip, which is when you feel paranoid, anxious, nervous or even terrified instead of euphoric. The only way to get over a bad trip is to wait it out. New users are often advised to have an experienced friend with them to guide them through the experience. Taking mushrooms can cause dizziness, nausea and other stomach problems, muscle weakness, loss of appetite and numbness. These symptoms subside as the trip comes to an end. Some mushroom users smoke marijuana to combat the nausea. Mushrooms aren't considered to be addictive, but tolerance builds up very quickly – taking mushrooms two days in a row often results in a less intense experience the second day, for example. There may be cross-tolerance with some other psychotropic drugs like LSD, mescaline and peyote, which means that taking one can build up tolerance for another [source: National Drug Intelligence Center]. So, are they dangerous? People with mental illnesses (diagnosed or not) have had their symptoms exacerbated through the use of mushrooms. There's no evidence of death caused by magic mushrooms; the amount that one would have to eat to cause death is hundreds of times greater than the normal dose. Death can result from taking misidentified mushrooms, however.

Types of Magic Mushrooms

Foraging for wild mushrooms is dicey. There are thousands of species, many with very similar features. Some toxic mushrooms can simply cause stomach problems, but others can cause organ failure and death. Hunting for any type of edible mushroom is generally best left to people who are very knowledgeable about mushroom identification. Even people who have been hunting mushrooms for decades have made mistakes. One part of the identification process is the creation of a spore print, which involves pressing the cap gill-side down onto a sheet of paper (usually both dark and white to see contrast) so that its spores are released.

There are dozens of species of mushroom within the genus Psilocybe. Most of them are on the small side   the average size is a 3-inch (7.6-centimeter) stalk and a 1-inch (2.5-centimeter) cap. When fresh, they usually have light grayish, yellowish or brownish stems with brown or brown-and-white caps and dark gills. We'll look at just a few of the most well-known varieties. Psilocybe cubensis is on the larger side as far as magic mushrooms go. It's also one of the most common. Called the common large Psilocybe, golden cap or Mexican mushroom, it has many different types. The cap is usually reddish brown, with a white or yellowish stem. When bruised or crushed, its sticky flesh often turns bluish. Some people consider this a definitive sign of finding a magic mushroom, but some toxic types of mushrooms bruise as well. It's usually found in moist, humid climates and grows on the dung of grazing animals like cattle.

Psilocybe semilanceata or liberty cap is a common psilocybin mushroom. In general, P. semilanceata is found in damp, grassy fields usually populated by cattle or sheep but unlike P. cubensis, it doesn't grow directly on the dung. It's a small mushroom, either light yellow or brown, with a very pointed cap. Another psilocybe mushroom, Psilocybe pelliculosa, is often mistaken for P. semilanceata, but its psychotropic properties are weaker.

Psilocybe baeocystis has a dark brown cap and brownish or yellowish stem when fresh. It can be found in fields in addition to growing on rotting logs, peat or mulch. Nicknames include potent Psilocybe, blue bell and bottle cap. So, do people who take magic mushrooms just pop a few into their mouths? Next, let's learn about what's considered a "dose" and the ways in which people consume magic mushrooms.

Mushroom Dosages: Feed Your Head

The dosage and intensity of magic mushrooms depends not only on the species, but where it was grown and how it has been handled. For example, there are several different strains of P. cubensis; Thai P. cubensis mushrooms are considered to be stronger and can result in a more intense high, while those found on the Gulf Coast are supposed to be produce a "mellower" high. The psylocybin content in the mushrooms also tends to deteriorate when they're dried, so people ingest more to compensate. Mushrooms are generally sold in the U.S. in eighths, meaning one-eighth of an ounce (3.5 grams), which usually costs around $35. The effects of magic mushrooms will always vary from person to person in addition to from mushroom to mushroom.

In general, people new to taking mushrooms are advised to start with roughly 1 gram (or less) of dried mushrooms (the equivalent of about one P. cubensis), wait an hour, and then, based on how they feel, decide whether to take more. Many people do simply chew on fresh or dried mushrooms, but they don't always taste good. Some magic mushrooms are described as having a floury taste, while others are sour or bitter – eating them with fruit such as strawberries can combat the flavor. People who really dislike the taste and texture come up with recipes for everything from smoothies to chili, although cooking the mushrooms for long periods of time will likely break down the psilocybin and result in a weaker psychotropic effect.

Magic mushrooms don't actually have to be eaten to feel their effects. They can be brewed into a mushroom tea by grinding them, steeping them in hot water and straining the resulting liquid. Proponents of this method claim that this has no impact on the intensity of the trip. Since alcohol and magic mushrooms are often used together, sometimes the mushrooms are soaked in rum or tequila and the liquid used in mixed drinks or simply drunk. People who have tripped on mushroom tea or extract say that they begin to feel the effects quicker than if they simply ate the mushroom. Finally, sometimes the dried mushrooms are ground and packed into gelatin capsules to create mushroom pills. This way, the taste and texture are avoided completely. Most people simply buy their magic mushrooms. As mentioned above, picking them in the wild is an option. However, some enterprising magic mushroom lovers cultivate their own at home.

Mycology: Growing Shrooms

The intensity of magic mushrooms can depend on where it was grown and how it has been handled.

Most mushrooms cultivators start with P. cubensis because it's the most common and the easiest to grow. There are several different ways to go about growing mushrooms, but we'll just look at one basic method. All methods begin with one important element: the spore. A spore grows into a single mushroom, and one mushroom can produce hundreds of thousands of spores.

Spore prints, in addition to being used for identification of wild mushrooms, can also be used to cultivate mushrooms. The dry spores on the print must be hydrated for use. Sterility is important in all aspects of mushroom growing; bacteria or mold can keep them from growing altogether, but may also result in contaminated mushrooms. Many mushroom growers purchase spore syringes (filled with spores and sterile water) from suppliers rather than make their own.

Other equipment includes a large plastic container, canning jars, a pressure cooker or canner, brown rice flour and vermiculite (a mineral gravel used in potting plants), as well as basic kitchen items. The brown rice flour is mixed with the water and vermiculite to create a loose, fluffy substrate cake, a nutrient-rich environment in which the mushroom spores will grow. The substrate is then put in the canning jars, which are sealed and sterilized using the pressure cooker or canner.

After the jars cool, the substrate is inoculated with the spore syringe through holes punched in the jars' lids. Then they must be incubated at a steady temperature of about 75 degrees Fahrenheit (23.9 degrees Celsius). The spores should begin to grow within a week and typically look like ropes of white fuzz called mycelium. If mold grows instead, or nothing happens, then something went wrong – you may have insufficiently sterilized your equipment, or perhaps you introduced contaminants during the inoculation process.

When the cakes are covered in mycelium, they are placed into the plastic container for fruiting. While in the container, the cakes must get light and a lot of humidity. If all goes well, mushrooms begin to grow after a week or two and are ready to pick when the caps begin to turn upward. Each cake can produce mushrooms for up to a month, usually in waves, called flushes. A single cake can produce dozens of mushrooms. They can rot pretty quickly, so mushrooms are usually refrigerated or dried to preserve them. Some avid growers graduate from basic techniques like these to what are called bulk growing methods. In bulk grows, the substrate may include materials like straw or manure, which must be pasteurized to prevent mold growth. Done properly, bulk growing techniques can produce hundreds or even thousands of mushrooms in one harvest. Growing mushrooms isn't all that expensive, but obtaining the spore prints or spore syringes can be difficult because it's not always legal to buy, sell or possess them. In the next section, we'll learn about the legality of magic mushrooms.

Magic Mushrooms and the Law

The legality of possessing, taking, growing or selling magic mushrooms greatly depends upon where you live. In the United States, psilocybin is a Schedule I drug under an amendment to the Controlled Substances Act called the Psychotropic Substances Act. This means that it has a high potential for abuse, has no currently accepted medical use and isn't safe for use even under a doctor's supervision. Since psilocybin is a psychotropic substance in magic mushrooms, this is usually interpreted to mean that the mushrooms themselves are illegal. However, since mushroom spores don't contain psilocybin, some have pointed to this as an ambiguity in the federal law.

Usually busts related to magic mushrooms occur under state law (unless they're in extremely large amounts) and most states ban possession of them. In recent years, though, cities and states have begun to reevaluate their stance on mushrooms. In 2019, Denver became the first city in the U.S. to decriminalize magic mushrooms. Santa Cruz and Oakland, California followed suit. With those victories in hand, mushroom legalization activists are hard at work in other states. Legislators in Oregon, California, and Iowa have introduced bills supporting mushroom decriminalization.

Possession and selling of fresh mushrooms and spores (dried mushrooms are almost always illegal) is still legal in many places around the world. But laws from nation to nation are wildly inconsistent. For example, until 2005, it was legal to sell fresh magic mushrooms in Great Britain; spore possession is still legal. The Netherlands, once known as a hotbed for drugs illegal elsewhere, banned the sale of dried mushrooms in 2001 and fresh mushrooms in 2008, but you're still allowed to be in possession of small amounts of "magic truffles," which refers to magic mushrooms that aren't quite fully developed, thereby skirting the law. Mexico bans mushrooms outright ... unless they're used for religious purposes. In Spain, mushrooms are decriminalized, but grow kits might not go over very well with the authorities.

In other countries, it may be legal to have them but not sell them. And in others, penalties for possession can be severe. In Indonesia, for instance, authorities sometime dole out death sentences for anyone who possess these kinds of substances. Other nations have zero interesting in policing or penalizing mushroom growers or users. In Jamaica, Bahamas and Brazil, for example, mushrooms are totally legal. Some countries, such as Mexico, make exceptions to bans on magic mushrooms when used by indigenous populations in religious ceremonies.

What to Know About Magic Mushroom Use

Magic mushrooms are wild or cultivated mushrooms that contain psilocybin, a naturally-occurring psychoactive and hallucinogenic compound. Psilocybin is considered one of the most well-known psychedelics, according to the Substance Abuse and Mental Health Services Administrations.

Psilocybin is classified as a Schedule I drug, meaning that has a high potential for misuse and has no currently accepted medical use in treatment in the United States. Although certain cultures have known to use the hallucinogenic properties of some mushrooms for centuries, psilocybin was first isolated in 1958 by Dr. Albert Hofmann, who also discovered lysergic acid diethylamide (LSD). Magic mushrooms are often prepared by drying and are eaten by being mixed into food or drinks, although some people eat freshly picked magic mushrooms. Also Known As: Magic mushrooms are also known as shrooms, mushies, blue meanies, golden tops, liberty caps, philosopher's stones, liberties, amani, and agaric.

Drug Class: Psilocybin is classified as a hallucinogen.

Common Side Effects: Magic mushrooms are known to cause nausea, yawning, feeling relaxed or drowsy, introspective experience, nervousness, paranoia, panic, hallucinations, and psychosis.

How to Recognize Shrooms

Mushrooms containing psilocybin look liked dried ordinary mushrooms with long, slender stems that are whitish-gray and dark brown caps with light brown or white in the center. Dried mushrooms are rusty brown with isolated areas of off-white. Magic mushrooms can be eaten, mixed with food, or brewed like tea for drinking. They can also be mixed with cannabis or tobacco and smoked. Liquid psilocybin is also available, which is the naturally occurring psychedelic drug found in liberty caps. The liquid is clear brown and comes in a small vial.

What Do Magic Mushrooms Do?

Magic mushrooms are hallucinogenic drugs, meaning they can cause you to see, hear, and feel sensations that seem real but are not. The effects of magic mushrooms, however, are highly variable and believed to be influenced by environmental factors. Shrooms have a long history of being associated with spiritual experiences and self-discovery. Many believe that naturally occurring drugs like magic mushrooms, weed, and mescaline are sacred herbs that enable people to attain superior spiritual states. Others take magic mushrooms to experience a sense of euphoria, connection, and a distorted sense of time.

The psilocybin found in shrooms is converted to psilocin in the body and is believed to influence serotonin levels in the brain, leading to altered and unusual perceptions. The effects take 20 to 40 minutes to begin and can last up to 6 hours the same amount of time it takes for psilocin to be metabolized and excreted. A number of factors influence the effects of magic mushrooms, including dosage, age, weight, personality, emotional state, environment, and history of mental illness.

WHAT THE EXPERTS SAY

While magic mushrooms are often sought out for a peaceful high, shrooms have been reported to induce anxiety, frightening hallucinations, paranoia, and confusion in some. In fact, most hospital admissions related to the use of magic mushrooms are connected to what is known colloquially as a "bad trip."

Off-Label or Recently Approved Uses

Magic mushrooms have been used for thousands of years for both spiritual and medicinal uses among indigenous people of America and Europe. In 2018, researchers from John Hopkins University recommended reclassification of the drug from Schedule I to Schedule IV in order to allow for medical use. Studies suggest that psilocybin can be used to treat cancer-related psychiatric distress, depression, anxiety, nicotine addiction, and substance use disorders.3

In 2019, Denver became the first city to decriminalize mushrooms. Oakland became the second city less than a month later. This does not mean that shrooms are legal but that the city is not permitted to "spend resources to impose criminal penalties" on people in possession of the drug.

Common Side Effects

All hallucinogens carry the risk of triggering mental and emotional problems and causing accidents while under the influence. Among adolescents, magic mushrooms are frequently taken in combination with alcohol and other drugs, increasing the psychological and physical risks. The amount of psilocybin and psilocin contained in any given magic mushroom is unknown, and mushrooms vary greatly in the amounts of psychoactive contents. This means it's very hard to tell the length, intensity, and type of "trip" someone will experience.

Consuming shrooms can result in a mild trip causing the user to feel relaxed or drowsy to a frightening experience, marked by hallucinations, delusions, and panic. In the worst-case scenario, magic mushrooms have even been known to cause convulsions.

Side effects of magic mushrooms can include both physical and mental effects.
Physical effects:
Dilated pupils

Drowsiness

Headaches

Increased heart rate, blood pressure, and temperature

Lack of coordination

Muscle weakness

Nausea

Yawning

Mental effects:
Distorted sense of time, place, and reality

Euphoria

Hallucinations (visual or auditory)

Having introspective (spiritual) experiences

Panic reactions

Paranoia

Psychosis

Nervousness

More research is needed on the long-term, lasting side effects of magic mushrooms but it has been reported that users can experience long-term changes in personality, as well as flashbacks long after taking mushrooms.

Since magic mushrooms look similar to poisonous mushrooms, poisoning is yet another potential risk of taking these drugs. Mushroom poisoning can cause severe illness, organ damage, and even death.

It's also common for magic mushroom products to be contaminated. A study of 886 samples alleged to be psilocybin mushrooms analyzed by Pharm Chem Street Drug Laboratory showed that only 252 (28%) were actually hallucinogenic, while 275 (31%) were regular store-bought mushrooms laced with LSD or phencyclidine (PCP), and 328 (37%) contained no drug at all.

Help for Mushroom Poisoning

If you suspect that you or someone you care about ate a poisonous mushroom, call poison control right. Don't wait for symptoms to occur. They are available 24 hours a day, seven days a week, 365 days a year.

Signs of Use

If your loved one is using shrooms, they may be nauseous or appear nervous or paranoid. In the case of drug use, it's always important to pay attention to any changes in sleeping and eating patterns as well as shifts in mood and personality and social activities.

Myths & Common Questions

There are many myths about magic mushrooms. Some people believe, for example, that magic mushrooms are "safer" and produce a "milder" trip than other hallucinogenics. In fact, in addition to their potential to poison anyone who takes them, magic mushrooms are just as unpredictable in their effects as other drugs. Some people have reported much more intense and frightening hallucinations on magic mushrooms than on LSD. Many people also confuse fly agaric mushrooms with psilocybin-containing mushrooms but they are not the same. Fly agaric mushrooms contain the psychoactive chemicals ibotenic acid and muscimol, which are known to cause twitching, drooling, sweating, dizziness, vomiting, and delirium.

Tolerance, Dependence, and Withdrawal

Like most drugs, the more you use magic mushrooms, the more tolerance you develop. Tolerance also develops quickly with regular use. This means that you need more of the drug to achieve the same effect.

Developing a tolerance can be especially risky with shrooms because consuming a large amount can result in overdose symptoms, which while not fatal, can include agitation, vomiting, diarrhea, muscle weakness, panic or paranoia, psychosis, and seizures.

How Long Does Psilocybin (Mushrooms) Stay in Your System?

The short-term effects of magic mushrooms typically wear off in 6 to 12 hours. But users can experience long-term changes in personality and flashbacks long after taking the drugs. The average half-life of psilocybin ranges from an hour to two, and it generally takes five to six half-lives for a substance to be eliminated from your system. The typical urine drug screening for employment does not test for psilocybin, but there are specific tests that can be ordered to test for the powerful hallucinogen. Like many other drugs, magic mushrooms can be found in hair follicles for up to 90 days.8

ADDICTION

Psilocybin is not addictive and does not lead to compulsive use. This is partly because the drug can cause an intense "trip." Plus, people can build a tolerance to psilocybin fairly quickly, making it hard to have any effect after several days of repeated use.

WITHDRAWAL

While users rarely report physical symptoms of withdrawal when they stop using the drug, some experience psychological effects, which may include depression.

HOW TO GET HELP

If you suspect your teen is experimenting or regularly using magic mushrooms, consider having a firm yet loving conversation with them about the risks of psychedelics, especially when combined with alcohol or other drugs. At this time, it's also important to emphasize that you are there to help and support them.

WHAT ARE MAGIC MUSHROOMS AND PSILOCYBIN?

What is psilocybin?

Psilocybin is a hallucinogenic substance people ingest from certain types of mushroom that grow in regions of Europe, South America, Mexico, and the United States. The mushrooms containing psilocybin are known as magic mushrooms. Psilocybin is a schedule-I controlled substance, meaning that it has a high potential for abuse and serves no legitimate medical purpose. Individuals use psilocybin as a recreational drug. It provides feelings of euphoria and sensory distortion that are common to hallucinogenic drugs, such as LSD. Although medical bodies do not consider psilocybin to be an addictive substance, users can experience disturbing hallucinations, anxiety, and panic from using the drug.

Fast facts on psilocybin

Psilocybin has both positive and negative physical and psychological effects.

Psilocybin is not naturally addictive.

The drug can trigger psychotic episodes.

Individuals with a family history of schizophrenia or early onset mental illness face an increased risk of an adverse psychiatric reaction to psilocybin.

WHAT IS PSILOCYBIN?

Psilocybin is a natural hallucinogen.

Psilocybin is a hallucinogen that works by activating serotonin receptors, most often in the prefrontal cortex. This part of the brain affects mood, cognition, and perception. Hallucinogens work in other regions of the brain that regulate arousal and panic responses. Psilocybin does not always cause active visual or auditory hallucinations. Instead, it distorts how some people that use the drug perceive objects and people already in their environment. The quantity of the drug, past experiences, and expectations of how the experience will take shape can all impact the effects of psilocybin. After the gut ingests and absorbs psilocybin, the body converts it to psilocyn. The hallucinogenic effects of psilocybin usually occur within 30 minutes of ingestion and last between 4 and 6 hours. In some individuals, the changes in sensory perception and thought patterns can last for several days. Mushrooms containing psilocybin are small and usually brown or tan. In the wild, people often mistake mushrooms containing psilocybin for any number of other mushrooms that are poisonous.

People usually consume psilocybin as a brewed tea or prepare it with a food item to mask its bitter taste. Manufacturers also crush dried mushrooms into a powder and prepare them in capsule form. Some people who consume these mushrooms cover them with chocolate.

The potency of a mushroom depends on:

The species

Origin

Growing conditions

Harvest period

Whether a person eats them fresh or dried

The amount of active ingredients in dried mushrooms is about 10 times higher than the amount found in their fresh counterparts.

Extent of use

In the U.S., the National Survey on Drug Use and Health (NSDUH) suggested that, between 2009 and 2015, around 8.5 percent of people reported using psilocybin at some point in their life.

When people use psilocybin, it is usually at dance clubs or in select groups of people seeking a transcendent spiritual experience. In medical settings, doctors have tested psilocybin for use in treating cluster headaches, end-stage cancer anxiety, depression, and other anxiety disorders. However, scientists have questioned its effectiveness and safety as a therapeutic measure.

Street names for psilocybin

Drug dealers rarely sell psilocybin under its real name. Instead, the drug may be sold as:

Magic mushrooms

Shrooms

Boomers

Zoomers

Mushies

Simple Simon

Little smoke

Sacred mushrooms

Purple passion

Mushroom soup

Cubes

Psilocybin as a treatment for depression

Discussions are on-going about whether psychological specialists can use psilocybin and similar hallucinogens as a treatment for depression. Two very recent studies have looked at psilocybin as a treatment. One study examined the ability of psilocybin to reduce depression symptoms without dulling emotions, and the other assessed the relationship between any positive therapeutic outcomes and the nature of psilocybin-induced hallucinations. While some researchers are looking into some therapeutic uses for psilocybin, they still, at present, regard psilocybin as unsafe and illegal.

Risks

People who have taken psilocybin in uncontrolled settings might engage in reckless behavior, such as driving while intoxicated. Some people may experience persistent, distressing alterations to the way they see the world. These effects are often visual and can last from anywhere from weeks to years after using the hallucinogen. Physicians now diagnose this condition as hallucinogen persisting perception disorder (HPPD), also known as a flashback. A flashback is a traumatic recall of an intensely upsetting experience. The recollection of this upsetting experience during hallucinogen use would be a bad trip, or a hallucination that takes a disturbing turn.

Some individuals experience more unpleasant effects than hallucinations, such as fear, agitation, confusion, delirium, psychosis, and syndromes that resemble schizophrenia, requiring a trip to the emergency room. In most cases, a doctor will treat these effects with medication, such as benzodiazepines. These effects often resolve in 6 to 8 hours as the effects of the drug wear off.

Finally, though the risk is small, some psilocybin users risk accidental poisoning from eating a poisonous mushroom by mistake. Symptoms of mushroom poisoning may include muscle spasms, confusion, and delirium. Visit an emergency room immediately if these symptoms occur. Because hallucinogenic and other poisonous mushrooms are common to most living environments, a person should regularly remove all mushrooms from areas where children are routinely present to prevent accidental consumption. Most accidental mushroom ingestion results in minor gastrointestinal illness, with only the most severe instances requiring medical attention.

Abuse potential

Psilocybin is not chemically addictive, and no physical symptoms occur after stopping use. However, regular use can cause an individual to become tolerant to the effects of psilocybin. Cross-tolerance also occurs with other drugs, including LSD and mescaline. People who use these drugs must wait at least several days between doses to experience the full effect. After several days of psilocybin use, individuals might possibly experience psychological withdrawal and have difficulty adjusting to reality.

Introduction to pain management

Pain management can be simple or complex, depending on the cause of the pain. An example of pain that is typically less complex would be nerve root irritation from a herniated disc with pain radiating down the leg. This condition can often be alleviated with an epidural steroid injection and physical therapy. Sometimes, however, the pain does not go away. This can require a wide variety of skills and techniques to treat the pain. These skills and techniques include:

Interventional procedures

Medication management

Physical therapy or chiropractic therapy

Psychological counseling and support

Acupuncture and other alternative therapies; and

Referral to other medical specialists

All of these skills and services are necessary because pain can involve many aspects of a person's daily life.

How is pain treatment guided?

The treatment of pain is guided by the history of the pain, its intensity, duration, aggravating and relieving conditions, and structures involved in causing the pain. In order for a structure to cause pain, it must have a nerve supply, be susceptible to injury, and stimulation of the structure should cause pain. The concept behind most interventional procedures for treating pain is that there is a specific structure in the body with nerves of sensation that is generating the pain. Pain management has a role in identifying the precise source of the problem and isolating the optimal treatment. Fluoroscopy is an X-ray guided viewing method. Fluoroscopy is often used to assist the doctor in precisely locating the injection so that the medication reaches the appropriate spot and only the appropriate spot. Ultrasound is also used to identify structures and guide injections.

What are the basic types of pain?

There are many sources of pain. One way of dividing these sources of pain is to divide them into two groups, nociceptive pain and neuropathic pain. How pain is treated depends in large part upon what type of pain it is.

Nociceptive pain

Examples of nociceptive pain are a cut or a broken bone. Tissue damage or injury initiates signals that are transferred through peripheral nerves to the brain via the spinal cord. Pain signals are modulated throughout the pathways. This is how we become aware that something is hurting.

Neuropathic pain

Neuropathic pain is pain caused by damage or disease that affects the nervous system. Sometimes there is no obvious source of pain, and this pain can occur spontaneously. Classic examples of this pain are shingles and diabetic peripheral neuropathy. It is pain that can occur after nerves are cut or after a stroke. Most back, leg, and arm pain is nociceptive pain. Nociceptive pain can be divided into two parts, radicular or somatic.

Radicular pain

Radicular pain is pain that stems from irritation of the nerve roots, for example, from a disc herniation. It goes down the leg or arm in the distribution of the nerve that exits from the nerve root at the spinal cord. Associated with radicular pain is radiculopathy, which is weakness, numbness, tingling or loss of reflexes in the distribution of the nerve.

Somatic pain

Somatic pain is pain limited to the back or thighs. The problem that doctors and patients face with back pain, is that after a patient goes to the doctor and has an appropriate history taken, a physical exam performed, and appropriate imaging studies (for example, X-rays, MRIs or CT scans), the doctor can only make an exact diagnosis a minority of the time. The cause of most back pain is not identified and is classifies as idiopathic. Three structures in the back which frequently cause back pain are the facet joints, the discs, and the sacroiliac joint. The facet joints are small joints in the back of the spine that provide stability and limit how far you can bend back or twist. The discs are the "shock absorbers" that are located between each of the bony building blocks (vertebrae) of the spine. The sacroiliac joint is a joint at the buttock area that serves in normal walking and helps to transfer weight from the upper body onto the legs. Fluoroscopically (x-ray) guided injections can help to determine from where pain is coming. Once the pain has been accurately diagnosed, it can be optimally treated.

Neuropathic pain includes:

Complex regional pain syndrome (CRPS), also called reflex sympathetic dystrophy;

Sympathetically maintained pain;

Fibromyalgia;

Interstitial cystitis; and

Irritable bowel syndrome.

Treatment of neuropathic pain

The various neuropathic pains can be difficult to treat. However, with careful diagnosis and often a combination of methods of treatments, there is an excellent chance of improving the pain and return of function.

Medications are a mainstay of treatment of neuropathic pain. In general, they work by influencing how pain information is handled by the body. Most pain information is filtered out by the central nervous system, usually at the level of the spinal cord. For example, if you are sitting in a chair, your peripheral nerves send the response to the pressure between your body and the chair to your nervous system. However, because that information serves no usual purpose, it is filtered out in the spinal cord. Many medications to treat neuropathic pain operate on this filtering process. The types of medications used for neuropathic pain include antidepressants, which influence the amount of serotonin or norepinephrine, and antiseizure medications, which act on various neurotransmitters, such as GABA and glycine. One of the most powerful tools in treating neuropathic pain is the spinal cord stimulator, which delivers tiny amounts of electrical energy directly onto the spine. Stimulation works by interrupting inappropriate pain information being sent up to the brain. It also creates a tingling in the pain extremity, which masks pain.

Other causes of pain include:

Headaches,

Facial pain,

Peripheral nerve pain,

Coccydynia,

Compression fractures,

Post-herpetic neuralgia,

Myofasciitis,

Torticollis,

Piriformis syndrome,

Plantar fasciitis,

Lateral epicondylitis, and

Cancer pain .

Headaches and facial pain, including a typical facial pain and trigeminal neuralgia.

Headaches are a major source of discomfort and lost productivity in the workplace. Many effective treatments exist for persisting headaches, including medication, biofeedback, injections and implants, depending upon the precise type of headache. Botox also provides a useful means of effectively and safely treating headaches. Atypical facial pain can be debilitating. Often times it can be treated by injections into local nerve tissue (such as the sphenopalatine ganglion).

Trigeminal neuralgia, also called tic douloureux, is a condition that most commonly causes very intense intermittent shooting pain in the face.

Peripheral nerve pain

Peripheral nerve pain, or neuropathy, can be debilitating. It can respond well to simple treatments such a trigger point injections with anesthetic medicines and cryoablation (an office based procedure which involves freezing the nerves). Examples of peripheral nerve pain include intercostal neuralgia, ilioinguinal neuroma, hypogastric neuroma, lateral femoral cutaneous nerve entrapment, interdigital neuroma and related nerve entrapments.

Coccydynia

Coccydynia is simply pain in the region on the tailbone, or coccyx. It can result from trauma or arise without apparent cause. The initial treatment is conservative, with oral pain relief medicines (analgesics). Oftentimes, the pain originates in the portion of the nervous system that we have no control of (involuntary or autonomic nervous system) and can respond to either a local anesthetic injection of the head of a nerve called Ganglion Impar, which is located below the coccyx or by medically destroying (ablating) the Ganglion Impar, usually using radiofrequency.

Compression fractures

Compression fractures of the bony building blocks (vertebral bodies) are common in the elderly as a result of osteoporosis, or loss of calcium in the bone. With less calcium, the bone becomes weak and can break. Like any fracture, compression fractures hurt. Like any fracture, they are treated by stabilization, in this case, by injecting cement into the bone in a procedure known as a vertebroplasty or kyphoplasty. Vertebroplasty is an effective way to treat the pain of compression fractures. Kyphoplasty uses a balloon to restore height to the compressed vertebral body.

Post-herpetic neuralgia

Post herpetic neuralgia (PHN) is a painful condition occurring after a bout of shingles. When we are young, we are almost all exposed to chickenpox, caused by the Herpes Zoster virus. Our immune system controls the virus, but it lives in a dormant state in the spinal cord. When we age, or become ill or stressed, the virus can reactivate and attack the infected nerve and adjacent skin. However, in this second attack, the body usually recognizes the Herpes Zoster virus and contains the pain to a localized area, along the course of one nerve. A patient may have the characteristic blisters, which normally heal. Sometimes, however, the Herpes Zoster virus damages the nerve, causing ongoing nerve pain that persists after the skin blisters from the shingles have healed.

The ideal way to treat the post herpetic neuralgia is to treat it before it sets in. Medications, such as acyclovir (Zovirax), steroids and injections such as sympathetic injections can help prevent the onset of PHN. After the pain is present, injections, local anesthetics, medications [duloxetine (Cymbalta), amitriptyline, (Elavil, Endep)] and pain medications or topical patches can be useful.

Myofasciitis and Torticollis

Myofasciitis (pain in the muscles, whether in the neck or back) often responds to conservative physical therapy treatments (for example, massage and exercise). If the pain persists, trigger point injections can be used. If the trigger point injections provide temporary relief, sometimes Botox injections can help. Botox, which is botulinum toxin, can relax the muscles for six or more months, with long-term relief of pain. It provides a safe, effective treatment for what can otherwise be a difficult, ongoing problem.

Torticollis is spasm of the muscles in the neck, forcing the sufferer to hold his or her neck tilted or rotated to the side. Botox is approved for treatment of this problem.

Piriformis Syndrome

The piriformis muscle goes from the hip to sacrum (tailbone). It is important in that the sciatic nerve passes through it. Piriformis syndrome is a spasm of the piriformis muscle. When the muscle goes into spasm, it can squeeze the sciatic nerve, causing pain going down the leg. Piriformis syndrome will usually respond to physical therapy.

When pain persists, local anesthetic and/or steroid injection can help. If the pain persists, injecting Botox or Myobloc, which are both botulinum toxins, into the muscle can provide effective, safe treatment.

Plantar fasciitis and lateral epicondylitis

Plantar fasciitis (heel pain) and lateral epicondylitis (tennis elbow) are two common pain problems. Treatment starts with conservative options, such as rest, non-steroidal anti-inflammatory medications, steroid injections, over-the counter pain medications, physical therapy and, for heel pain, shoe inserts.

If the pain lasts for more than six months, Extracorporeal Shockwave Treatment is an effective, FDA approved treatment. Extracorporeal shockwave treatment is not recommended for pregnant women, children, anyone with a pacemaker, anyone on anti-coagulant therapy or anyone with a history of bleeding problems.

Cancer pain

Cancer pain can arise from many different causes, including the cancer itself, compression of a nerve or other body part, fractures or treatment of the cancer. There are many techniques to assist with treating the various pains from cancer, including medications and injections. In particular, medical destruction of nerve tissue (ablative therapies) and the use of pumps surgically placed into the body to deliver pain medication into the subarachnoid space can be used. Pain pumps deliver medication that is targeted to pain receptors on the spinal cord. The advantage to the cancer patient is chronic pain control with decreased side effects.

Microdosing Mushrooms: Does It Help with Chronic Pain?

In the 16th century, the Aztecs used it to stimulate mystical experiences. They called it 'teonanacatl,' or sacred mushroom. In the modern age, workers in Silicon Valley have made microdosing popular. They use it as a productivity edge in uber-competitive work environment. You might know this mystical substance as "magic mushrooms." You may not know that 21st-century scientists are exploring the medical potential of a method of use called 'microdosing.

A Brief History of Microdosing Mushrooms

History of Microdosing Mushrooms Microdosing is not a new idea. The pharmaceutical industry uses microdosing to learn about a drug's pharmacokinetics. In the 1960s, psychologist and researcher James Fadiman was experimenting with using psychedelics as medicine. His research ended when recreational use of hallucinogens became popular and the government stopped funding the experiments.

At that time, the research on psilocybin was showing exciting promise in two areas: substance abuse and end-of-life anxiety and depression.

In the early 2000s, there was new interest in psilocybin, the active compound in "magic mushrooms," as a medical treatment. The Food and Drug Administration (FDA) gave the study of psychedelic drugs "breakthrough status." Dr. Fadiman and others could now resume research in psychedelics as medicine. Since its early use in Silicon Valley, more people began microdosing mushrooms. Many consider it a productivity hack because it can increase focus, cognitive ability, and creativity.

NOTE: At this time, the hallucinogen in magic mushrooms is a schedule I drug (meaning it has no accepted medical use). It is still illegal in most places. Our intent in writing this article is to inform our readers of research that may have future benefits for chronic pain sufferers.

What Is Microdosing, and How Can It Help Pain Patients?

Microdosing is the use of a tiny dose of a psychedelic substance (one-tenth of the usual "trip dose") to improve cognitive abilities, concentration, or creativity without experiencing an altered level of consciousness. In the case of magic mushrooms, the active compound is psilocybin, a hallucinogen produced by many types of fungi. While pain relief isn't the most common reason people give for microdosing psilocybin, some say it helps with certain types of pain. There are few clinical trials on the microdosing of psilocybin for pain. Still, there are reports that it can be helpful with phantom limb pain and cluster headaches. Another potential benefit for chronic pain sufferers is the treatment of pain-induced psychiatric symptoms. Psilocybin can elevate mood and reduce symptoms of anxiety and treatment-resistant depression. It may help to break the pain-depression-pain cycle that debilitates many chronic pain sufferers.

Microdosing for Mental Health Conditions

The effect of microdosing can be twofold for people with chronic pain. While it helps with long-term pain like cluster headaches, it also works as a psychedelic serotonin agonist (PSA). PSAs work on the neurologic pathways of the brain. They create new links that allow parts of the brain that don't normally communicate, talk to each other and create new thoughts and experiences. This reorganizing of brain pathways may be the key to how psilocybin improves anxiety and depression symptoms: It may disrupt dysfunctional pathways as it creates new ones. The effects of this reorganization can have long-term results. Full-dose studies found that psilocybin reduced symptoms of cancer-related anxiety (with one dose) and treatment-resistant depression (with two spaced doses) for six months and three months, respectively. In all, seven clinical trials found that psilocybin use caused reductions in psychiatric rating scores or improved response and remission rates. What's more, psilocybin may be protective against suicidality.

Microdosing Mushrooms for Addiction

The studies mentioned above found psilocybin to also be a promising treatment for alcohol and tobacco addiction with increased abstinence rates and no severe adverse reactions. The mechanism that makes psilocybin a potential treatment for anxiety and depression may work in the same way to reduce addictive behaviors. In another study, most participants reported significantly decreased use of alcohol, caffeine, cannabis, illicit substances, and psychiatric medications. Researchers concluded that psilocybin microdosing warrants more research on its potential to treat substance use disorders. Microdosing Mushrooms for Addiction. This could be great news for chronic pain sufferers who form addictions by self-medicating to decrease pain.

Risks and Side Effects of Psilocybin

For all its potential benefits, psilocybin also carries risks. The most common side effects are headaches that are not severe or disabling and mood lability. Both are more likely to occur with higher doses, however. Other reported side effects include dizziness, nausea, muscle weakness, numbness, and loss of appetite.

The Future of Mushroom Microdosing

As discussed above, in 2018, the Food and Drug Administration (FDA) approved a clinical trial of psilocybin as a treatment for depression. Since then, Johns Hopkins University has established a Center for Psychedelic and Consciousness Research. For now, though, mushrooms are still illegal in the US, though three cities have decriminalized them: Denver, Colorado; Oakland, California; and Santa Cruz, California. The state of Oregon is working toward doing the same, but the coronavirus pandemic has slowed down their progress. In the meantime, Johns Hopkins uses synthetic psilocybin in pill form in their clinical trials. A synthetic form of the drug would make therapeutic dosing accurate and predictable for use as a pharmaceutical.

CONCLUSION

Psilocybin is known to increase mood, concentration, creativity, and productivity, but research is still in the early stages. While we know that it helps with cluster headaches and phantom limb pain, researchers have only scratched the surface of its potential to treat pain.

Still, some researchers have found mushroom microdosing to be safe and non-addictive, and it may be an effective treatment for other conditions that can contribute to chronic pain, such as anxiety, depression, and substance abuse.